THE COMPLETE HIGH TRIGLYCERIDE COOKBOOK FOR NEWLY DIAGNOSED

1600 DAYS OF NUTRITIOUS RECIPES FOR A HEALTHY HEART AND LOWERING HIGH TRIGLYCERIDES

KAREN EDMONDS

1

Copyright © 2024 Karen Edmonds

TABLE OF CONTENT

INTRODUCTION

If you have recently been diagnosed with excessive triglycerides, it is understandable to be concerned about your health and question how to make good changes. The Complete High Triglyceride Cookbook is prepared to be a reliable partner on your quest to optimal heart health.

This cookbook is an excellent resource for individuals who have recently been diagnosed, since it gives practical and tasty solutions for managing and lowering triglyceride levels via mindful eating. High triglycerides can raise your risk of developing heart disease, thus this cookbook strives to provide you with easy, yet delectable dishes that prioritise heart-healthy components.

These pages provide a range of meals that are both healthful and satisfying. From energising breakfast alternatives like Greek Yoghurt Parfait with Berries to nourishing meals like Baked Cod with Lemon and

Herbs, each recipe is carefully prepared to benefit your cardiovascular health. Whole meals, lean proteins, and good fats are emphasised as key components of a heart-healthy lifestyle.

Even if you are not a seasoned chef, this cookbook will help you prepare meals that are both beneficial for your heart and tasty. The Complete High Triglyceride Cookbook is your go-to reference for choosing healthy food choices to build a healthier heart. Allow this cookbook to serve as the foundation for a tasty and heart-conscious culinary adventure as you navigate and embrace a healthy lifestyle.

CHAPTER 1

Understanding Triglycerides

Triglycerides are a form of fat in the blood that play an important role in energy storage. They are generated by the breakdown of lipids and carbohydrates in the diet. Triglycerides circulate in the bloodstream and are stored in fat cells, ready to be turned back into energy as needed. While they play an important role in metabolism, maintaining balance is critical for general health.

The Effects of High Triglycerides on Health

Triglyceride levels that are too high might offer serious health hazards, especially to the cardiovascular system. This section of the conversation delves into the repercussions of excessive triglycerides, such as its link to heart disease, stroke, and other cardiovascular disorders. It also addresses the relationship between triglycerides, cholesterol levels, and the total lipid profile.

Importance of Heart-Healthy Diet

A heart-healthy diet is more than simply a delicious choice; it is an essential component of total well-being, particularly for cardiovascular health. This section emphasises the need of including dietary choices that enhance heart health and, especially, assist regulate triglyceride levels.

Reducing cardiovascular risk:

A heart-healthy diet helps to reduce the risk factors for cardiovascular disease. Individuals who eat more nutrient-dense meals can improve their cholesterol, blood pressure, and, most importantly, triglyceride levels.

Managing triglycerides and cholesterol:

The dietary options presented in the cookbook are intended to precisely address high triglycerides. Individuals may actively regulate their lipid profile by eating foods high in omega-3 fatty acids, soluble fibre, and antioxidants, which promote a balance of good (HDL) and bad (LDL) cholesterol.

Supporting overall well-being:

A heart-healthy diet benefits both cardiovascular and general health. Nutrient-dense meals provide the body with critical vitamins, minerals, and antioxidants that are necessary for a variety of physical processes, including immune support and skin and organ health.

Weight Management:

Maintaining a healthy weight is crucial for heart health. The cookbook promotes mindful eating, emphasising portion management and nutrient density. This not only helps with weight control but also prevents obesity-related issues that might harm the heart.

Sustainable Lifestyle Changes:

Embracing a heart-healthy diet is a long-term lifestyle decision. This section encourages readers to think of dietary changes as a long-term commitment to their health, stressing the concept that tiny, consistent improvements can result in major advantages over time.

By understanding the significance of a heart-healthy diet, readers are empowered to make educated decisions that go beyond triglyceride management, supporting a more holistic approach to cardiovascular wellness.

CHAPTER 2

Triglyceride-friendly basics

Understanding the principles of a triglyceride-friendly diet is essential for making long-term, meaningful adjustments to your eating habits. This section is a practical reference, giving important suggestions and information to help you make smart food choices.

Healthy fats 101:

Distinguish between good fats (avocado, almonds, and olive oil) and bad fats (saturated and trans- from butter, cheese, fatty cuts of meat). Learn how to include good fats into your diet while reducing detrimental ones to improve heart health.

Omega-3 Powerhouses:

Investigate the effects of omega-3 fatty acids in controlling triglyceride levels. Discover high-quality sources such as fatty fish (salmon, mackerel), flaxseeds, and walnuts, and discover how to include them into your meals.

Fiber-Rich Choices:

Understand how soluble fibre can help decrease triglycerides and improve overall heart health. Identify high-fiber foods such as oats, beans, and fruits, and learn simple recipes to make fibre consumption a fun part of your daily routine.

Lean Proteins for Balance:

To keep your diet balanced, choose lean protein sources including poultry, fish, and plant-based proteins. Learn about portion sizes and cooking strategies that keep protein consumption healthy while avoiding excessive saturated fats.

Smart carbohydrate selection:

Embrace complex carbs such as whole grains, vegetables, and legumes while limiting processed carbohydrates. Investigate the effects of carbs on triglyceride levels and find appealing alternatives to refined grains.

Portion-Control Strategies:

Learn the art of portion control to avoid overeating and aid with weight management. Learn visual clues and practical techniques to keep your meals balanced without feeling deprived.

Mindful Eating Habits:

Create mindful eating habits that emphasise savouring each mouthful and paying attention to hunger and fullness indicators. This method promotes a healthy connection with food and can help to improve overall dietary choices.

Establishing a firm foundation in triglyceride-friendly essentials will provide you with the information and skills you need to confidently navigate your dietary choices, encouraging both heart health and pleasant eating experiences.

Essential Kitchen Tools for Healthy Cooking

Quality Chef Knife:

A sharp, high-quality chef's knife is required for rapid and accurate cutting of fruits, vegetables, and lean meats. Invest in a quality knife to make dinner preparation easier.

Non-stick Cookware:

Choose non-stick pans to reduce the need for excessive cooking oils or fats. This guarantees that your meals are low in dangerous saturated fats and promotes quick cleanup.

Steam Basket:

A steamer basket is a flexible instrument for cooking vegetables, cereals, and meats while preserving important nutrients. Steaming retains food's inherent flavours and textures.

Food Processor:

A food processor is a versatile instrument that may assist with chopping, slicing, and mixing. Use it to make healthful dips, sauces, and dishes that use nuts.

Blender:

A high-quality blender is ideal for creating healthy smoothies, soups, and sauces. It allows you to include a range of fruits and vegetables to your diet in a simple and delightful way.

Measuring cup and spoon:

Accurate portioning is essential for eating a balanced meal. Invest in accurate measuring cups and spoons to guarantee you are using the correct amounts of components.

Digital Food Scale:

A digital food scale allows you to accurately measure ingredients, particularly when it comes to portion management. This tool is very beneficial for balancing fats and carbs in your meals.

How to Read Food Labels

Serving Size Awareness:

Understand the portion size shown on the label and compare it to how much you regularly consume. Adjusting portion sizes based on these suggestions helps you manage calories and nutrients more effectively.

Check the Total Fat Content:

Concentrate on the kind and amount of fats in the product. Choose meals with minimal saturated and trans fat content, and prioritise healthy fats such as monounsaturated and polyunsaturated fats.

Evaluate Sugar Content:

Be wary of any added sugars in items. Choose low-sugar goods and sweeten your food with natural sweeteners or entire fruits.

Look for whole grains:

Identify entire grains in the ingredient list, such as whole wheat, brown rice, or oatmeal. Whole grains support a heart-healthy diet by delivering critical minerals and fibre.

Sodium Awareness:

Check the salt levels in packaged goods. High salt consumption can cause high blood pressure, which is a risk factor for heart disease.

Check for fibre:

Choose meals with a greater fibre content. Fibre assists digestion, regulates blood sugar levels, and promotes a sensation of fullness.

Ingredient List Inspection:

Pay close attention to the ingredient list to detect and avoid artificial additives, preservatives, and harmful hydrogenated oils. Choose items with simple and identifiable components.

With these important kitchen equipment and an awareness of how to read food labels, you will be well equipped to produce nutritious, triglyceride-friendly meals and make smart grocery shopping decisions

STAY HEALTHY AND HAPPY

CHAPTER 3: BREAKFAST BOOSTERS

Energizing Oatmeal with Berries

Ingredients:

- 1/2 cup rolled oats
- 1 cup of milk (dairy or plant-based almond or skim mik)
- 1/2 teaspoon of vanilla extract
- 1 tablespoon of chia seeds
- 1/2 cup of mixed berries (strawberries, blueberries, raspberries)
- 1 tablespoon of honey or maple syrup (optional)
- 1 tablespoon of chopped nuts (almonds, walnuts) for garnish
- Fresh mint leaves for garnish

Preparation:

Combine Oats and Milk:

- In a saucepan, add together the rolled oats and milk. Bring to a moderate simmer over medium heat, stirring periodically to keep from sticking.

Add vanilla extract and chia seeds:

- Once the oats have begun to absorb the liquid, add the vanilla essence and chia seeds. Continue to toss and cook the oats until they reach the desired consistency.

Fold in berries:

- Gently fold in the mixed berries, leaving a few for topping. The heat will soften the berries, infusing the muesli with their natural sweetness.

Sweeten (optional):

- If desired, sprinkle honey or maple syrup over the muesli for extra sweetness. Adjust to your taste preferences.

Serve:

- Spoon the energising muesli into a bowl. Top with the saved berries, chopped almonds, and fresh mint leaves for a blast of flavour and texture.

Enjoy:

- Dive into a hearty bowl of energising muesli, savouring the creamy oats, sweet berries and crunchy almonds.

Nutritional Value (Approximate, per serving):

Calories: 300-350 kcal

Protein: 10g

Fat: 10g (including healthy fats from chia seeds and nuts)

Carbohydrates: 45g

Dietary Fibre: 8g

Sugar: 15g (mainly from natural sugars in berries)

Calcium: 300mg

Iron: 3mg

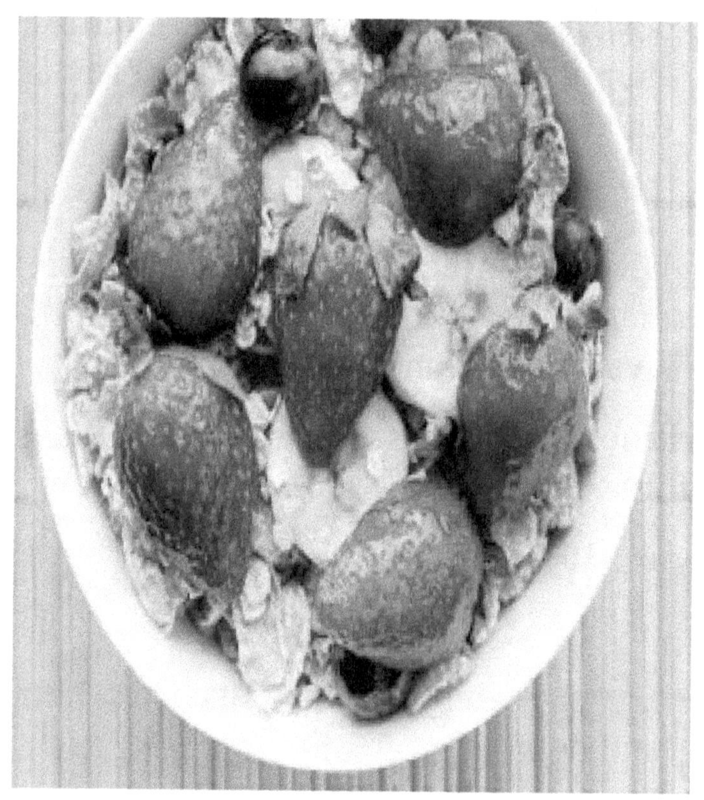

Notes

Your

Observation

Greek Yogurt Parfait with Nuts and Seeds

Ingredients:

- 1 cup of Greek yogurt (unsweetened)
- 1 tablespoon of honey or maple syrup (optional, for sweetness)
- 1/2 cup of granola (choose a low-sugar, whole-grain variety)
- 2 tablespoons of mixed nuts (almonds, walnuts) chopped
- 1 tablespoon of mixed seeds (chia seeds, flaxseeds, pumpkin seeds)
- 1/2 cup fresh berries (strawberries, blueberries, raspberries)
- 1 teaspoon of pure vanilla extract
- A sprinkle of cinnamon (optional)
- Fresh mint leaves for garnish

Preparation:

Prepare Greek Yogurt Base:

- Combine the Greek yoghurt, honey or maple syrup (if using), and vanilla extract in a bowl. Adjust the sweetness to your taste.

Layering:

- In a glass or dish, begin by putting a dollop of the Greek yoghurt mixture on the bottom.

Add Granola Layer:

- Sprinkle oats over the Greek yoghurt. This provides crunch and whole-grain *deliciousness to the parfait.*

Nut and Seed Layer:

- Add a layer of chopped nuts and seeds. These include healthy fats, protein, and an additional dosage of nutrients.

Repeat Layers:

- Repeat layering until you reach the top of the glass or bowl. Serve with a dollop of Greek yoghurt on top.

Top with berries:

- Garnish the parfait with an abundance of fresh berries. The natural sweetness and brilliant colours improve the overall flavour and look.

Optional: Sprinkle with cinnamon:

- Sprinkle some cinnamon on top for extra flavour. Cinnamon balances the sweetness and provides warmth to the parfait.

Garnish with mint leaves:

- Garnish the parfait with fresh mint leaves for a punch of flavour.

Serve and enjoy:

- Serve the Greek Yoghurt Parfait with Nuts & Seeds right away, enabling the layers to mix together for a delicious blend of textures and flavours.

Nutritional Value (Approximate, per serving):

Calories: 350-400 kcal

Protein: 20g

Fat: 15g (including healthy fats from nuts and seeds)

Carbohydrates: 40g

Dietary Fibre: 7g

Sugar: 18g (mainly from natural sugars in yogurt and berries)

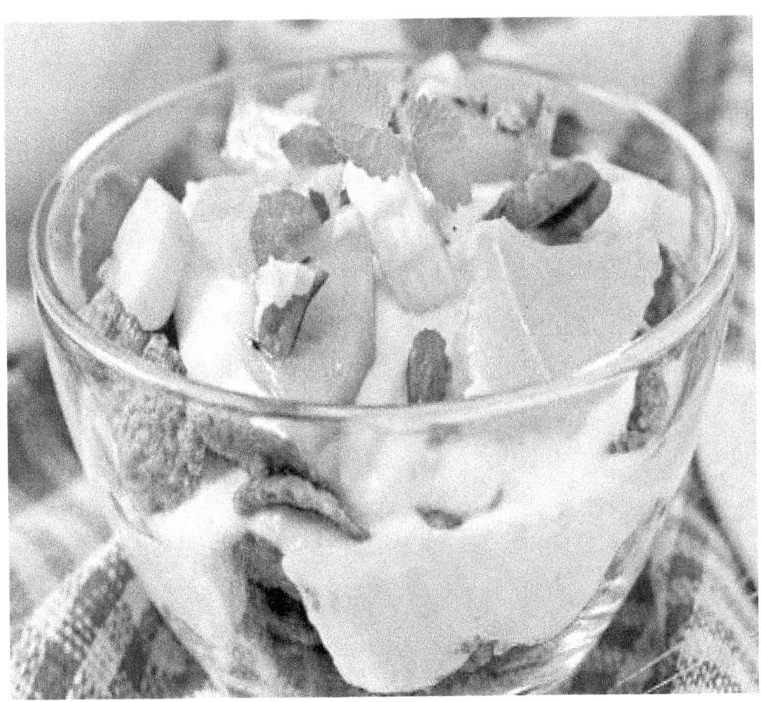

Notes

Your

Observation

Avocado and Tomato Breakfast Wrap

Ingredients:

- 1 whole-grain or whole-wheat tortilla
- 1 ripe avocado, sliced
- 1 medium-sized tomato, chopped
- 2 eggs
- Salt and pepper to taste
- Optional toppings: salsa, hot sauce, cilantro, or feta cheese
- Cooking spray or a small amount of olive oil for frying

Preparation:

Prepare Avocado and Tomato:

- Cut the avocado and tomatoes into thin, uniform slices. Season the tomato slices with a touch of salt and pepper.

Scramble the eggs:

- In a mixing dish, whisk the eggs and season with salt and pepper. Heat a nonstick pan over medium heat and coat lightly with cooking spray or olive oil. Pour the eggs into the skillet and scramble until done.

Warm the tortilla:

- Put the tortilla in a separate, dry skillet over medium heat. Warm it for 10-15 seconds on each side until it is flexible.

Assemble the Wrap:

- Place the hot tortilla on a flat surface. In the centre of the tortilla, place the sliced avocado, tomato, and scrambled eggs.

Add optional toppings:

- Drizzle salsa or spicy sauce over the stuffing to enhance the flavour. Sprinkle with cilantro or crumbled feta cheese, if preferred.

Fold & Roll:

- Fold the tortilla's edges inside, then roll it up firmly from the bottom to form a wrap.

Slice and serve:

- If desired, cut the wrap in half diagonally for better handling. Arrange the slices on a dish, seam side down.

Enjoy:

- Indulge in this scrumptious Avocado and Tomato Breakfast Wrap, which has creamy avocado, juicy tomato, and fluffy scrambled eggs.

Nutritional Value (Approximate, per serving):

Calories: 400-450 kcal

Protein: 15g

Fat: 25g (including healthy fats from avocado and eggs)

Carbohydrates: 35g

Dietary Fibre: 10g

Sugar: 3g (from natural sugars in tomatoes)

Notes

**Your
Observation**

CHAPTER 4: WHOLESOME LUNCHES

Quinoa Salad with Grilled Chicken and Vegetables

Ingredients:

For the Salad:

- 1 cup of quinoa, washed
- 2 cups of water or vegetable broth (for cooking quinoa)
- 1 pound boneless, skinless chicken breasts
- 1 tablespoon of olive oil
- Salt and pepper to taste
- 1 cup of cherry tomatoes, halved
- 1 cucumber, diced
- 1 red bell pepper, chopped
- 1/2 red onion, finely chopped
- 1/4 cup feta cheese, crumbled (optional)

- Fresh parsley or cilantro, chopped (for garnish)

For the Dressing:

- 3 tablespoons of extra virgin olive oil
- 2 tablespoons of balsamic vinegar
- 1 teaspoon of Dijon mustard
- 1 clove of minced garlic
- Salt and pepper to taste

Preparation:

Cook Quinoa:

- Rinse the quinoa under cool water. In a saucepan, mix the quinoa with the water or vegetable broth. Bring to a boil, then lower the heat, cover, and simmer for 15-20 minutes, or until the quinoa is cooked and the water is absorbed. Fluff with a fork and allow to cool.

Grill chicken:

- Preheat your grill or grill pan. Season chicken breasts with salt and pepper after rubbing with olive oil. Grill for 6-8 minutes per side, or until well done. Let the chicken rest for a few minutes before slicing it into thin pieces.

Prepare vegetables:

- In a large mixing bowl, add the cooked quinoa, grilled chicken strips, cherry tomatoes, cucumber, red bell pepper, red onion, and feta cheese, if desired.

Make the dressing:

- In a small mixing bowl, combine the extra virgin olive oil, balsamic vinegar, Dijon mustard, minced garlic, salt, and pepper. Adjust the seasoning to your liking.

Prepare the Salad:

- Pour the dressing over the quinoa-chicken combination. Gently mix the ingredients until well covered with the dressing.

Garnish and serve:

- Top the quinoa salad with fresh parsley or cilantro. Serve immediately or chill for a bit to let the flavours mingle.

Enjoy:

- Enjoy this nutritious Quinoa Salad with Grilled Chicken and vegetables, which combines protein-packed quinoa, grilled chicken, and a rainbow of fresh, crisp vegetables.

Nutritional Value (Approximate, per serving):

Calories: 400-450 kcal

Protein: 30g

Fat: 18g (including healthy fats from olive oil and chicken)

Carbohydrates: 35g

Dietary Fibre: 6g

Sugar: 4g (from natural sugars in vegetables)

Notes

Your

Observation

Ingredients:

- 1 cup of dried green or brown lentils, washed and drained
- 1 tablespoon of olive oil
- 1 large onion, chopped
- 2 carrots, peeled and diced
- 2 celery stalks, diced
- 3 cloves of minced garlic
- 1 teaspoon of ground cumin
- 1 teaspoon of ground coriander
- 1/2 teaspoon of smoked paprika
- 1 can (14 ounces) diced tomatoes, undrained
- 6 cups of vegetable broth
- 2 bay leaves
- Salt and pepper to taste
- 2 cups of kale or spinach, chopped
- 1 lemon, juiced
- Fresh parsley, chopped (for garnish)

Preparation:

Prepare Lentils:

- Heat the olive oil over medium heat in a big soup pot. Add the diced onions, carrots, and celery. Sauté the vegetables for 5-7 minutes, or until tender.

Add Aromatics and Spices:

- Stir in the minced garlic, ground cumin, ground coriander, and smoked paprika. Sauté for a further 1-2 minutes, until aromatic.

Incorporate tomatoes and lentils:

- Add the chopped tomatoes with juices and the rinsed lentils to the saucepan. Stir to mix.

Pour in vegetable broth:

- Pour in the vegetable broth and add the bay leaves. Bring the soup to a boil, then lower the heat, cover, and cook for 20-25 minutes, or until the lentils are cooked.

Season and add greens:

- Season the soup with salt and pepper, to taste. Add the chopped kale or spinach and simmer for another 5 minutes, or until the greens have wilted.

Finish with lemon juice:

- Squeeze the juice of one lemon into the soup and adjust the acidity to your taste. Discard the bay leaves.

Serve and garnish:

- Ladle the lentil and vegetable soup into dishes. Garnish with fresh parsley to enhance freshness and flavour.

Enjoy:

- This healthful and hearty lentil and vegetable soup may be eaten alone or with a slice of whole-grain bread.

Nutritional Value (Approximate, per serving):

Calories: 250-300 kcal

Protein: 14g

Fat: 5g (including healthy fats from olive oil)

Carbohydrates: 45g

Dietary Fibre: 15g

Sugar: 8g (from natural sugars in vegetables)

Notes

Your

Observation

Ingredients:

For the Salad:

- 2 cups of fresh baby spinach leaves, washed and dried
- 6 ounces of grilled or baked salmon fillet, flaked
- 1 cup of cherry tomatoes, halved
- 1 cucumber, sliced
- 1/4 red onion, finely sliced
- 1/4 cup of feta cheese, crumbled
- 1/4 cup of Kalamata olives, pitted and sliced (optional)
- 1/4 cup of pine nuts, toasted

For the Lemon Dill Vinaigrette:

- 3 tablespoons of extra-virgin olive oil
- 2 tablespoons of fresh lemon juice
- 1 teaspoon of Dijon mustard
- 1 clove of minced garlic
- 1 tablespoon of fresh dill, cut

- Salt and pepper to taste

Preparation:

Prepare the Salad Base:

- In a big salad bowl, mix together the fresh baby spinach, flaked salmon, cherry tomatoes, cucumber slices, red onion, feta cheese, and Kalamata olives, if using.

Make the lemon dill vinaigrette:

- In a small mixing bowl, combine the extra virgin olive oil, fresh lemon juice, Dijon mustard, minced garlic, cut fresh dill, salt, and pepper. Adjust the seasoning to your liking.

Drizzle dressing over the salad:

- Drizzle the lemon-dill vinaigrette over the salad components. Toss carefully to evenly coat the salad in dressing.

Toast pine nuts:

- Toast the pine nuts in a dry pan over medium heat until they are golden brown. Take cautious not to burn them.

Add toasted pine nuts:

- To add crunch and flavour, sprinkle roasted pine nuts over the salad.

Serve immediately:

- Serve the Spinach and Salmon Salad immediately, making sure it is well-dressed and the flavours are bright.

Enjoy:

- This delicious and protein-packed Spinach and Salmon Salad is an excellent lunch or dinner option.

Nutritional Value (Approximate, per serving):

Calories: 400-450 kcal

Protein: 25g

Fat: 30g (including healthy fats from olive oil and salmon)

Carbohydrates: 15g

Dietary Fibre: 4g

Sugar: 5g (from natural sugars in vegetables)

Notes

Your

Observation

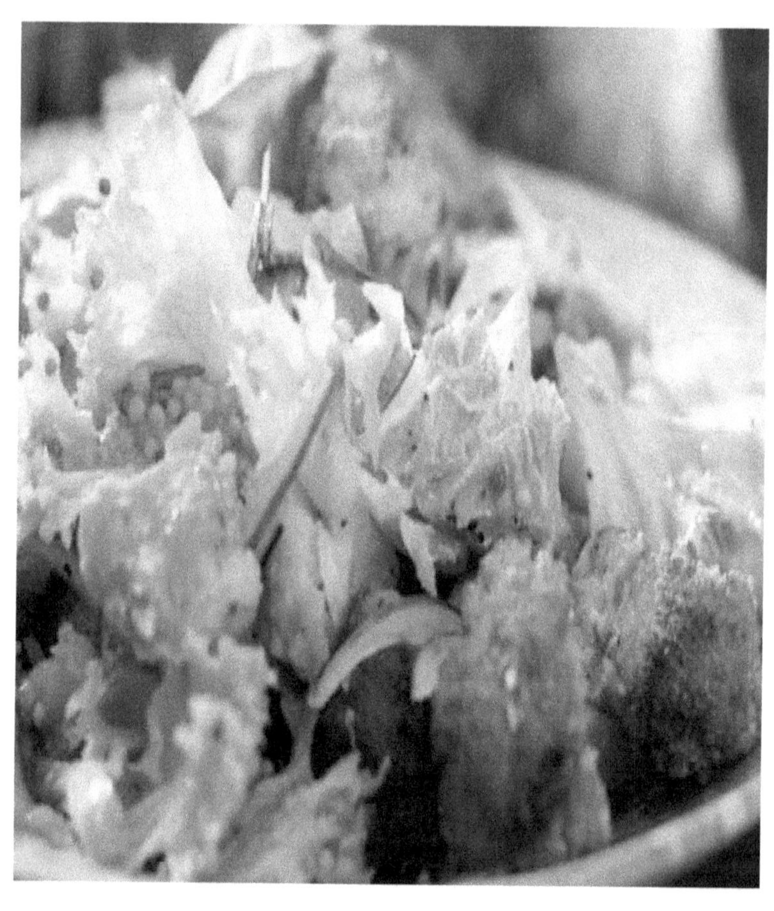

CHAPTER 5: NUTRIENT-PACKED DINNERS

Baked Cod with Lemon and Herbs

Ingredients:

- 4 cod fillets (about 6 ounces each), skinless
- 2 tablespoons of olive oil
- 2 tablespoons of fresh lemon juice
- 2 cloves of minced garlic
- 1 teaspoon of dried oregano
- 1 teaspoon of dried thyme
- 1 teaspoon of fresh parsley, cut
- 1/2 teaspoon of paprika
- Salt and pepper to taste
- Lemon slices for garnish
- Fresh parsley for garnish

Preparation:

Preheat the Oven:

- Preheat the oven to 400 °F (200 °C).
  Line a baking dish with parchment
  paper or gently oil it.

Prepare the cod fillets:

- Pat the cod fillets dry with a paper
  towel. Place them in the prepared
  baking dish.

Make the lemon-herb marinade:

- In a small mixing bowl, combine olive
  oil, fresh lemon juice, minced garlic,
  dried oregano, dried thyme, chopped
  parsley, paprika, salt, and pepper.

Marinate the cod:

- Pour the lemon-herb marinade over the
  cod fillets and make sure they are
  uniformly covered. Allow the fish to
  marinade for at least 15-20 minutes to
  fully absorb the flavours.

Bake the cod:

- Bake the cod fillets in the preheated oven for 15-20 minutes, or until they are opaque and readily flaked with a fork. The cooking time might vary depending on the thickness of the fillets.

Garnish and serve:

- Garnish the baked fish with lemon slices and fresh parsley for a pop of colour and flavour.

Serve immediately:

- Serve the Baked Cod with Lemon and Herbs right away, complemented by your favourite side dishes such as steamed vegetables, quinoa, or a fresh salad.

Enjoy:

- Enjoy this light and tasty meal, with the delicate taste of cod enhanced by the zesty lemon and fragrant herbs.

Nutritional Value (Approximate, per serving):

Calories: 250-300 kcal

Protein: 30g

Fat: 12g (including healthy fats from olive oil)

Carbohydrates: 2g

Dietary Fibre: 1g

Sugar: 0g (from natural sources)

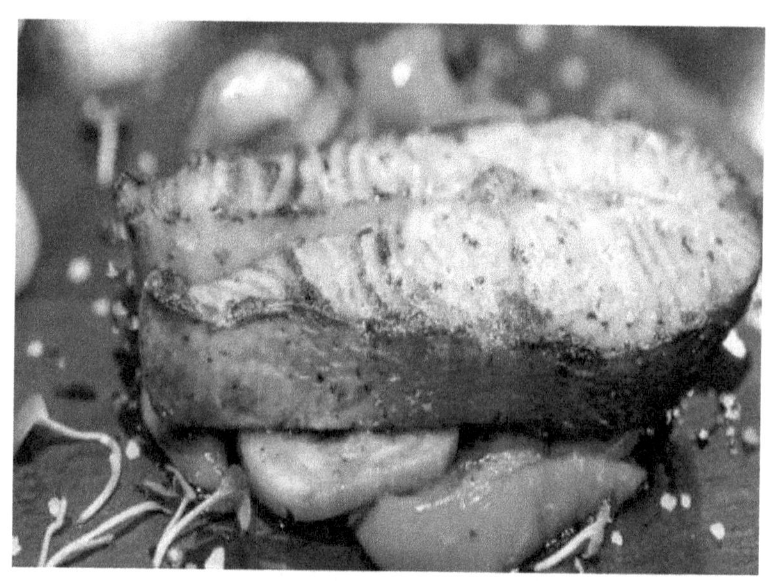

Notes

Your

Observation

Chickpea and Vegetable Stir-Fry

Ingredients:

- 1 can of (15 ounces) chickpeas, washed and drained
- 2 tablespoons of olive oil
- 2 cloves of minced garlic
- 1 onion, finely sliced
- 1 bell pepper (any color), thinly sliced
- 2 carrots, julienned or thinly sliced
- 1 cup of broccoli florets
- 1 cup of snow peas, trimmed
- 1 zucchini, sliced
- 1 teaspoon of grated ginger
- 2 tablespoons of soy sauce (or tamari for gluten-free option)
- 1 tablespoon of rice vinegar
- 1 tablespoon of honey or maple syrup
- 1 tablespoon of sesame oil
- 2 green onions, sliced (for garnish)
- Sesame seeds (for garnish)
- Cooked rice or quinoa, for serving

Preparation:

Prepare Ingredients:

- Rinse and drain the chickpeas. Prepare all vegetables by slicing, chopping, and julienning as directed.

Make the stir-fry sauce:

- Combine the soy sauce, rice vinegar, honey, maple syrup, and sesame oil in a small mixing bowl. Set aside.

Stir-Fried Vegetables:

- Heat the olive oil in a large pan or wok over medium-high heat. Sauté minced garlic and grated ginger for about 30 seconds, until aromatic.
- Add the cut onion and bell pepper to the skillet. Stir-fry for 2-3 minutes, or until they begin to soften.

Add remaining vegetables:

- Add the julienned carrots, broccoli florets, snow peas, and sliced zucchini to the skillet. Continue to stir-fry for another 3-4 minutes, or until the vegetables are soft and crisp.

Add chickpeas and sauce:

- Add the drained chickpeas to the skillet, along with the stir-fry sauce. Stir carefully to evenly coat the vegetables and chickpeas in the sauce.

Cook and finish:

- Cook for another 2-3 minutes, stirring regularly, until everything is well cooked and the flavours have melded together.

Garnish and serve:

- To add flavour and texture to the Chickpea and Vegetable Stir-Fry, garnish with sliced green onions and sesame seeds.

Serve over rice or quinoa:

- Serve the stir-fry hot over cooked rice or quinoa, which will provide a healthful and filling substrate for the aromatic veggies and chickpeas.

Enjoy:

- This healthy and colourful Chickpea and Vegetable Stir-Fry is a tasty and nourishing dinner full of protein, fibre, and critical elements.

Nutritional Value (Approximate, per serving, excluding rice/quinoa):

Calories: 250-300 kcal

Protein: 10g

Fat: 10g (including healthy fats from olive oil and sesame oil)

Carbohydrates: 30g

Dietary Fibre: 8g

Sugar: 8g (from natural sources and honey/maple syrup)

Notes

Your

Observation

Ingredients:

- 1 lb of ground turkey
- 1 tablespoon of olive oil
- 1 big onion, diced
- 3 cloves of minced garlic
- 1 bell pepper (any color), diced
- 1 big sweet potato, peeled and diced
- 1 can of (15 ounces) black beans, rinsed and drained
- 1 can of (15 ounces) kidney beans, rinsed and drained
- 1 can of (14 ounces) diced tomatoes, undrained
- 1 can (6 ounces) tomato paste
- 3 cups of low-sodium chicken or vegetable broth
- 2 teaspoons of chili powder
- 1 teaspoon of ground cumin
- 1 teaspoon of smoked paprika
- 1/2 teaspoon of ground cinnamon
- Salt and pepper to taste

- Optional toppings: shredded cheese, sliced green onions, Greek yogurt or sour cream, chopped cilantro

Preparation:

Ground Turkey:

- Heat the olive oil over medium heat in a large saucepan. Add the ground turkey and sauté until browned, breaking it up with a spoon as it cooks.

Sauté Aromatics:

- Add the diced onion, minced garlic, and diced bell pepper to the saucepan. Sauté the vegetables for 3-4 minutes, until they are softened.

Add sweet potato:

- Add the cubed sweet potato and simmer for another 5 minutes.

Combine beans and tomatoes:

- Add the black beans, kidney beans, chopped tomatoes, and tomato paste to the saucepan. Stir well to mix.

Season the chilli:

- Pour in the vegetable or chicken broth. Combine the chilli powder, ground cumin, smoked paprika, ground cinnamon, salt, and pepper. Stir to mix all of the ingredients.

Simmer:

- Bring the chilli to a boil, then lower to a low heat, cover, and cook for 20-25 minutes, or until the sweet potatoes are cooked.

Adjust seasoning:

- Taste and adjust the seasoning, adding more salt or spices as needed.

Serve:

- Ladle the Sweet Potato and Turkey Chilli into bowls. Optional toppings include shredded cheese, sliced green onions, a dollop of Greek yoghurt or sour cream, and chopped cilantro.

Enjoy:

- Enjoy this warm and tasty Sweet Potato and Turkey Chilli, a protein-rich dish with healthful ingredients.

Nutritional Value (Approximate, per serving):

Calories: 350-400 kcal

Protein: 25g

Fat: 10g (including healthy fats from olive oil and turkey)

Carbohydrates: 45g

Dietary Fibre: 12g

Sugar: 8g (from natural sources)

Notes

Your

Observation

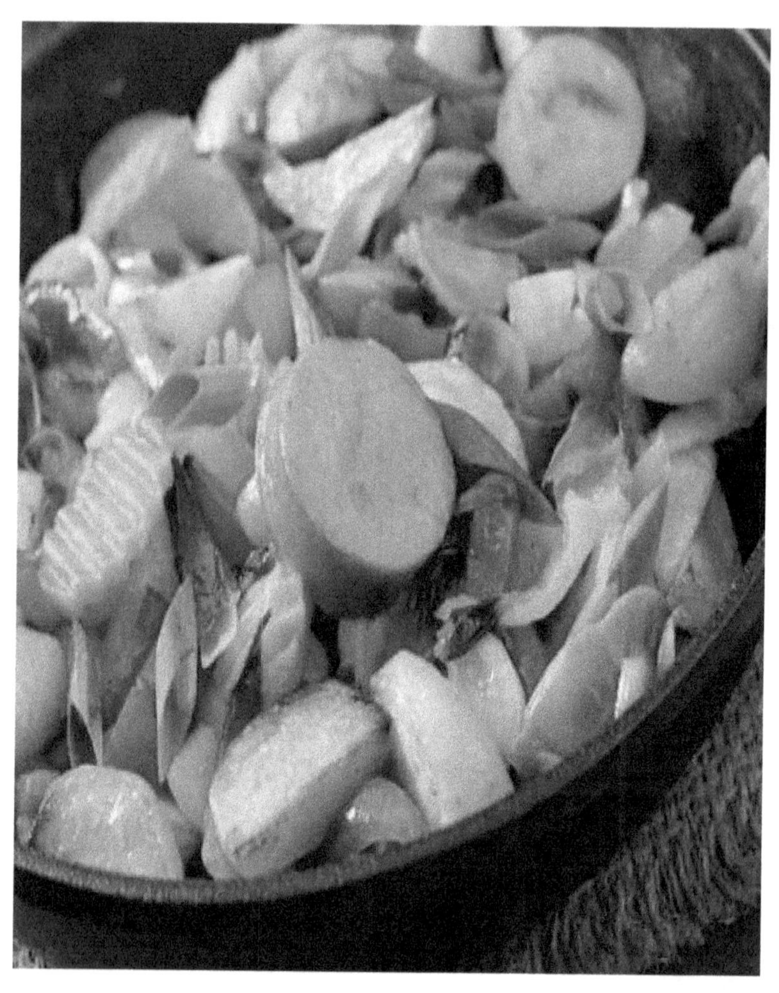

CHAPTER 6: SNACK IDEAS

Almond and Berry Smoothie

Ingredients:

- 1 cup of mixed berries (strawberries, blueberries, raspberries)
- 1 banana, peeled and sliced
- 1/4 cup of almonds, preferably soaked overnight
- 1 cup of almond milk (unsweetened)
- 1 tablespoon of almond butter
- 1 tablespoon of chia seeds (optional, for extra texture)
- 1 teaspoon of honey or maple syrup (optional, for extra sweetness)
- Ice cubes (optional)

Preparation:

Soak Almonds (Optional):

- If the almonds have not been soaked overnight, simply soak them in hot water for 15-20 minutes to soften.

Prepare Ingredients:

- Wash the mixed berries, then slice the banana.

Blend almonds:

- Combine the soaked almonds, almond milk, and almond butter in a blender. Blend until the almonds are well mixed and the mixture is smooth.

Add berries and bananas:

- Add the mixed berries and cut banana to the blender. Blend until all of the ingredients are fully mixed.

Incorporate chia seeds:

- If using chia seeds, place them in the blender and pulse briefly to integrate them into the smoothie.

Sweeten to taste:

- If you want the smoothie to be sweeter, add honey or maple syrup. Blend briefly to blend.

Optional: Add ice cubes:

- If you want your smoothie colder and thicker, add a handful of ice cubes and mix until smooth.

Serve immediately:

- Pour the almond and berry smoothie into a glass and serve immediately.

Garnish (optional):

- To enhance visual appeal, garnish with a few whole berries or a sprinkling of chopped almonds.

Enjoy:

- Enjoy the refreshing and nutrient-dense Almond and Berry Smoothie as a wonderful breakfast or snack.

Nutritional Value (Approximate):

Calories: 300-350 kcal

Protein: 8g

Fat: 20g (including healthy fats from almonds and almond butter)

Carbohydrates: 30g

Dietary Fibre: 8g

Sugar: 15g (from natural sugars in fruits)

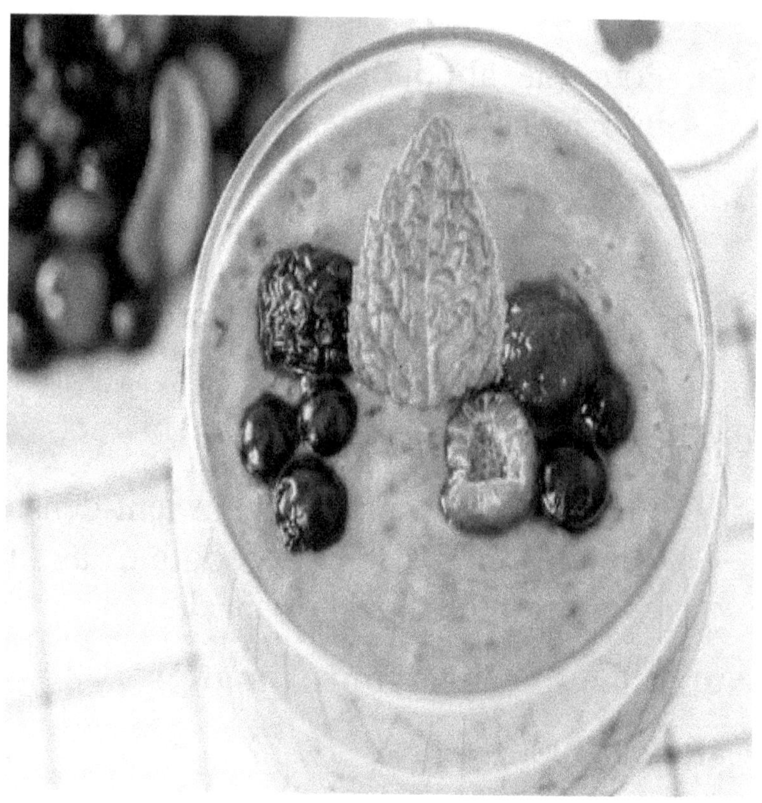

Notes

Your

Observation

Roasted Chickpeas with Spices

Ingredients:

- 2 cans of (15 ounces each) chickpeas, rinsed and drained
- 2 tablespoons of olive oil
- 1 teaspoon of ground cumin
- 1 teaspoon of smoked paprika
- 1/2 teaspoon of ground coriander
- 1/2 teaspoon of garlic powder
- 1/2 teaspoon of onion powder
- 1/4 teaspoon of cayenne pepper (adjust to taste for spiciness)
- Salt and pepper to taste

Preparation:

Preheat the Oven:

- Preheat the oven to 400 °F (200 °C).

Dry chickpeas:

- Using a paper towel, pat dry the drained chickpeas. The drier they are, the crisper they will become when roasted.

Season chickpeas:

- Combine the chickpeas, olive oil, ground cumin, smoked paprika, ground coriander, garlic powder, onion powder, cayenne pepper, salt, and pepper in a mixing bowl. Ensure that the chickpeas are uniformly covered with the spice mixture.

Spread on a baking sheet:

- Place the seasoned chickpeas in a single layer on a baking pan. Make sure they are not too packed so that they can roast evenly.

Roast in the oven:

- Roast the chickpeas in a preheated oven for 25-30 minutes, until golden brown and crispy. Shake the baking sheet halfway through to achieve an even roast.

Cool and serve:

- Let the roasted chickpeas cool slightly before serving. They will continue to crisp as they cool.

Store:

- If you have any leftovers (which are incredibly addicting), keep them in an airtight container. They are best eaten within a day or two for optimal crispiness.

Enjoy:

- Spiced Roasted Chickpeas are a crispy and savoury snack on their own, but they are also great in salads, soups, and as a yoghurt topping.

Variations:

Herb Variation: Try various herbs like rosemary, thyme, or oregano.

- For a cheesy touch, sprinkle grated Parmesan cheese over the chickpeas in the final few minutes of roasting.

Nutritional Value (Approximate, per serving):

Calories: 150-200 kcal

Protein: 7g

Fat: 7g (including healthy fats from olive oil)

Carbohydrates: 20g

Dietary Fibre: 6g

Sugar: 2g

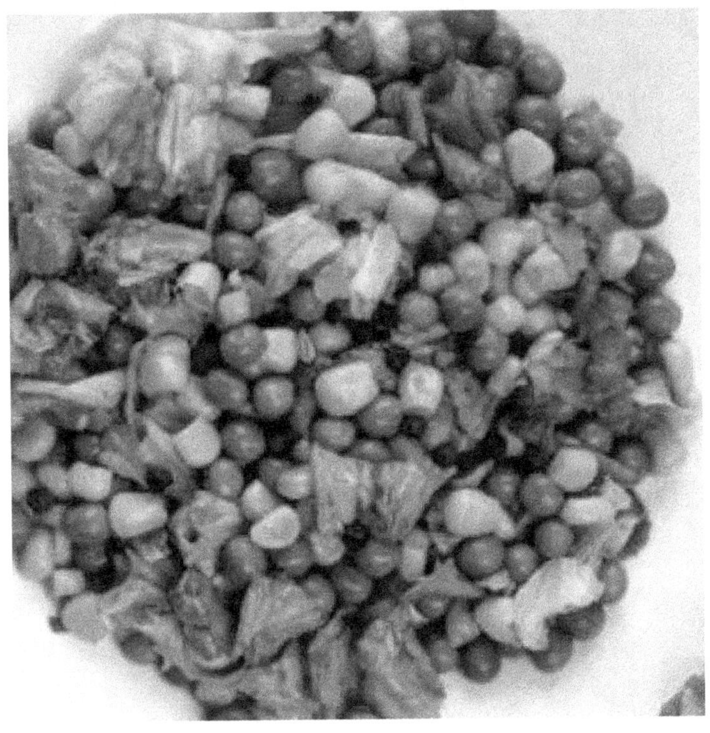

Notes

Your

Observation

Fresh Fruit Salsa with Cinnamon Pita Chips

Fresh Fruit Salsa with Cinnamon Pita Chips

Ingredients:

For the Fresh Fruit Salsa:

- 1 cup of diced fresh strawberries
- 1 cup of chopped fresh mango
- 1 cup of chopped pineapple
- 1/2 cup of diced kiwi
- 1/4 cup of finely chopped fresh mint leaves
- 1 tablespoon of honey or maple syrup
- 1 tablespoon of fresh lime juice

For the Cinnamon Pita Chips:

- 4 whole wheat pita bread rounds
- 2 tablespoons of olive oil
- 2 tablespoons of granulated sugar
- 1 teaspoon of ground cinnamon

Preparation:

Fresh Fruit Salsa:

Prepare Fruits:

- Wash, peel, and dice the strawberries, mangoes, pineapple, and kiwis.

Combine Ingredients:

- In a big mixing basin, carefully incorporate the diced fruits and finely chopped mint leaves.

Add sweetener and citrus:

- Drizzle some honey or maple syrup over the fruit combination. Squeeze some fresh lime juice on top. Gently toss the fruits to provide a uniform coating.

Chill:

- Cover the bowl with plastic wrap and chill the fruit salsa for at least 30 minutes to enable the flavours to combine.

Cinnamon pita chips:

Preheat the Oven:

- Preheat the oven to 350°F (175° C).

Prepare pita bread:

- Divide each pita bread round into wedges or triangles.

Make the Cinnamon Sugar Mixture:

- In a separate bowl, combine the granulated sugar and ground cinnamon to make the cinnamon sugar mixture.

Brush with olive oil:

- Place the pita wedges on a baking pan. Lightly brush each slice with olive oil.

Sprinkle cinnamon sugar:

- Sprinkle the cinnamon sugar mixture over the greased pita wedges, making sure it is evenly distributed.

Bake:

- Bake the pita chips in a preheated oven for 10-12 minutes, or until golden brown and crispy. Keep an eye on them to avoid burning.

Cool:

- Let the cinnamon pita chips cool fully on a wire rack.

Serve:

- *Fresh Fruit Salsa:* Serve chilled in a dish to highlight the brilliant colours and pleasant flavours.
- *Cinnamon Pita Chips:* Arrange cooled Cinnamon Pita Chips over a bowl of fruit salsa for a delicious and crunchy complement.

Enjoy:

- Enjoy this Fresh Fruit Salsa with Cinnamon Pita Chips as a tasty and nutritious snack or a refreshing appetiser at parties.

Nutritional Value (Approximate, per serving):

Calories: 200-250 kcal (including salsa and chips)

Protein: 3g

Fat: 7g (including healthy fats from olive oil)

Carbohydrates: 40g

Dietary Fibre: 6g

Sugar: 20g (from natural sugars in fruits and added sweetener)

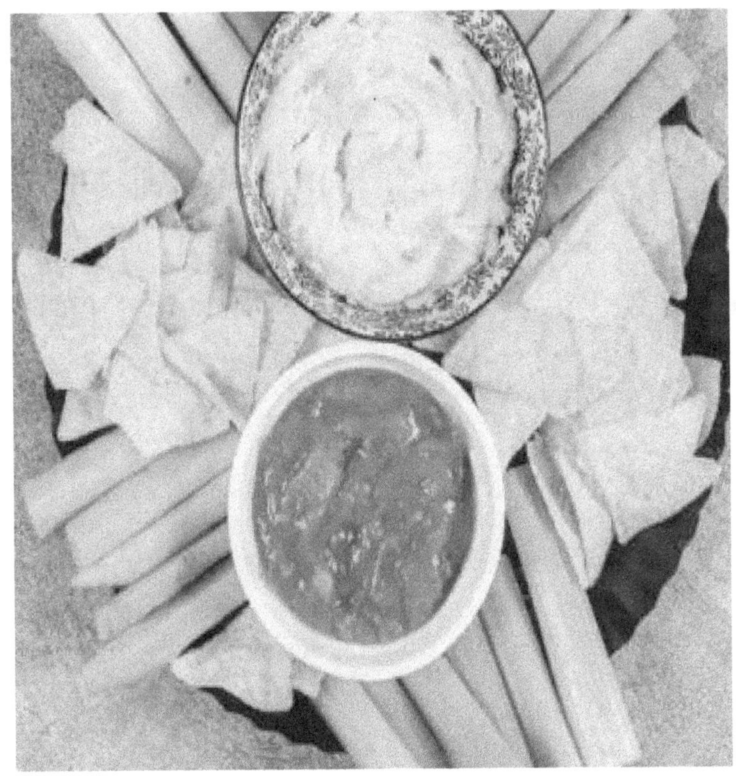

Notes

Your

Observation

CHAPTER 7: SATISFYING SIDES

Quinoa and Vegetable Stuffed Peppers

Ingredients:

- 4 large bell peppers, halved and seeds removed
- 1 cup of quinoa, rinsed
- 2 cups of vegetable broth or water
- 1 tablespoon of olive oil
- 1 onion, finely chopped
- 2 cloves of minced garlic
- 1 zucchini, diced
- 1 yellow squash, diced
- 1 carrot, grated
- 1 cup of cherry tomatoes, halved
- 1 cup of black beans, cooked and drained
- 1 teaspoon of ground cumin

- 1 teaspoon of paprika
- Salt and pepper to taste
- 1 cup of shredded cheese (cheddar, mozzarella, or your choice)
- Fresh parsley or cilantro for garnish (optional)

Preparation:

Preheat the oven:

- Preheat the oven to 375°F (190° C).

Prepare Quinoa:

- Mix the quinoa and vegetable broth/water in a saucepan. Bring to a boil, then lower to a low heat, cover, and simmer for 15-20 minutes, or until the quinoa is cooked and the liquid has been absorbed. Fluff with a fork. Place aside.

Prepare bell peppers:

- Cut the bell peppers in half lengthwise, then remove the seeds and membranes. Put them in a baking dish.

Sauté vegetables:

- Heat the olive oil over medium heat in a big skillet. Sauté chopped onion and garlic until transparent.

Add zucchini, squash and carrots:

- Add the chopped zucchini, yellow squash and shredded carrot to the pan. Cook for 5-7 minutes, until the veggies are soft.

Stir in the tomatoes and black beans:

- Stir in the halved cherry tomatoes and cooked black beans. Cook for another 2–3 minutes.

Season the mixture:

- Season the vegetables with ground cumin, paprika, salt, and pepper. Adjust the seasoning to your liking.

Combine Quinoa with Vegetables:

- Combine the cooked quinoa with the veggie mixture. Stir well to properly distribute the ingredients.

Stuff the peppers:

- Fill each bell pepper half with the quinoa and vegetable mixture, gently pushing down.

Top with cheese:

- Sprinkle the filled peppers with shredded cheese, being sure to cover the tops equally.

Bake:

- Bake in the preheated oven for 25-30 minutes, or until the peppers are soft and the cheese has melted and turned golden.

Garnish and serve:

- Garnish with fresh parsley or cilantro if preferred. Serve the Quinoa and Vegetable Stuffed Peppers hot.

Enjoy:

- Enjoy this nutritious and savoury dinner that combines the nutrition of quinoa, colourful veggies, and melty cheese.

Nutritional Value (Approximate, per serving):

Calories: 300-350 kcal

Protein: 12g

Fat: 10g (including healthy fats from olive oil and cheese)

Carbohydrates: 45g

Dietary Fibre: 8g

Sugar: 8g (from natural sugars in vegetables)

Notes

Your

Observation

Garlic and Herb Roasted Sweet Potatoes

Ingredients:

- 3 big of sweet potatoes, peeled and cut into bite-sized cubes
- 3 tablespoons of olive oil
- 4 cloves of minced garlic
- 1 teaspoon of dried rosemary
- 1 teaspoon of dried thyme
- 1 teaspoon of dried oregano
- Salt and pepper to taste
- Fresh parsley for garnish (optional)

Preparation:

Preheat the Oven:

- Preheat your oven to 400°F (200°C).

Prepare Sweet Potatoes:

- Peel and chop the sweet potatoes into bite-sized cubes.

Make a garlic and herb mixture:

- Combine olive oil, minced garlic, dried rosemary, thyme, oregano, salt, and pepper in a small mixing bowl.

Coat sweet potatoes:

- Put the sweet potato cubes in a big basin. Pour the garlic and herb mixture over the sweet potatoes, making sure they are thoroughly covered.

Spread on a baking sheet:

- Place the coated sweet potato cubes in a single layer on a baking sheet. Make sure they are not too packed so that they can roast evenly.

Roast in the oven:

- Roast the sweet potatoes in a preheated oven for 25-30 minutes, until golden brown and soft. Flip them midway during the cooking period to ensure equal roasting.

Garnish and serve:

- Once the sweet potatoes have been perfectly roasted, take them from the oven. Garnish with fresh parsley if preferred.

Serve immediately:

- Serve the Garlic and Herb Roasted Sweet Potatoes right away as a tasty and savoury side dish.

Enjoy:

- These flavorful and herb-infused roasted sweet potatoes make an excellent addition to your favourite dishes.

Nutritional Value (Approximate, per serving):

Calories: 200-250 kcal

Protein: 2g

Fat: 10g (including healthy fats from olive oil)

Carbohydrates: 30g

Dietary Fiber: 5g

Sugar: 6g (from natural sugars in sweet potatoes)

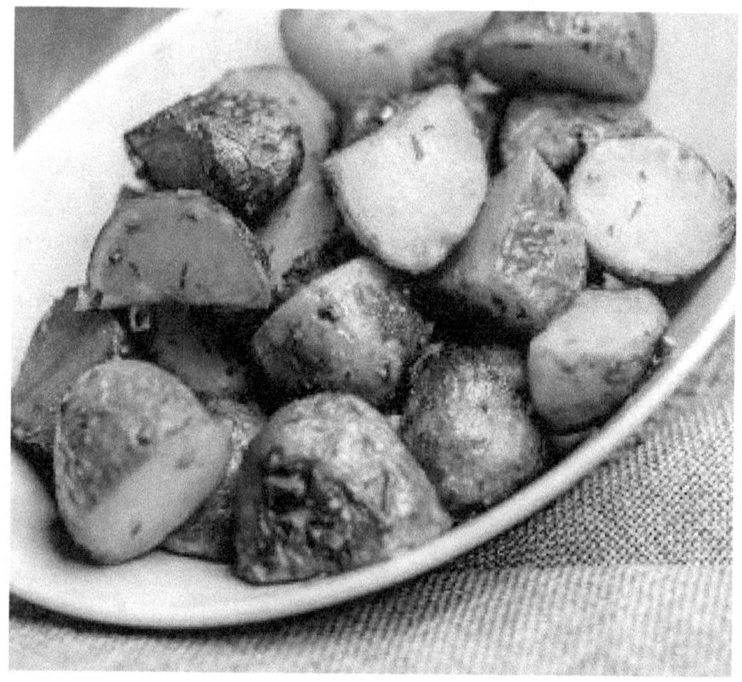

Notes

Your

Observation

Steamed Broccoli with Lemon Zest

Ingredients:

- 1 bunch of fresh broccoli, washed and cut into florets
- Zest of 1 lemon
- 2 tablespoons of olive oil
- 2 cloves of minced garlic
- Salt and pepper to taste
- Lemon wedges for serving (optional)

Preparation:

Prepare Broccoli:

- Wash the broccoli very well before cutting it into bite-size florets.

Steam broccoli:

- Place a steamer basket in a saucepan filled with a little water. Place the broccoli florets into the steamer basket. Cover the saucepan and steam for 5-7 minutes, or until the broccoli is brilliant green and soft but still crisp.

Prepare lemon zest:

- While the broccoli is cooking, use a zester or fine grater to zest the lemon. Make careful to zest just the exterior, yellow part of the lemon, not the bitter white pith.

Sauté garlic:

- In a small pan, heat the olive oil over medium heat. Sauté the minced garlic for 1-2 minutes, or until aromatic. Take care not to brown the garlic.

Combine the broccoli, lemon zest, and garlic:

- Once the broccoli has been cooked, transfer it to a serving basin. Drizzle the sautéed garlic and olive oil over the steaming broccoli. Sprinkle some lemon zest on top.

Season and toss:

- Season the broccoli with salt and pepper, to taste. Gently toss the broccoli to ensure that the lemon zest and garlic are evenly coated.

Serve:

- Serve the Steamed Broccoli with Lemon Zest immediately, garnished with more lemon wedges if preferred.

Enjoy:

- Enjoy easy and refreshing side dish that highlights the natural flavours of broccoli while enhancing them with the citrus brightness of lemon.

Nutritional Value (Approximate, per serving):

Calories: 80-100 kcal

Protein: 3g

Fat: 6g (including healthy fats from olive oil)

Carbohydrates: 8g

Dietary Fiber: 3g

Sugar: 2g (from natural sugars in broccoli)

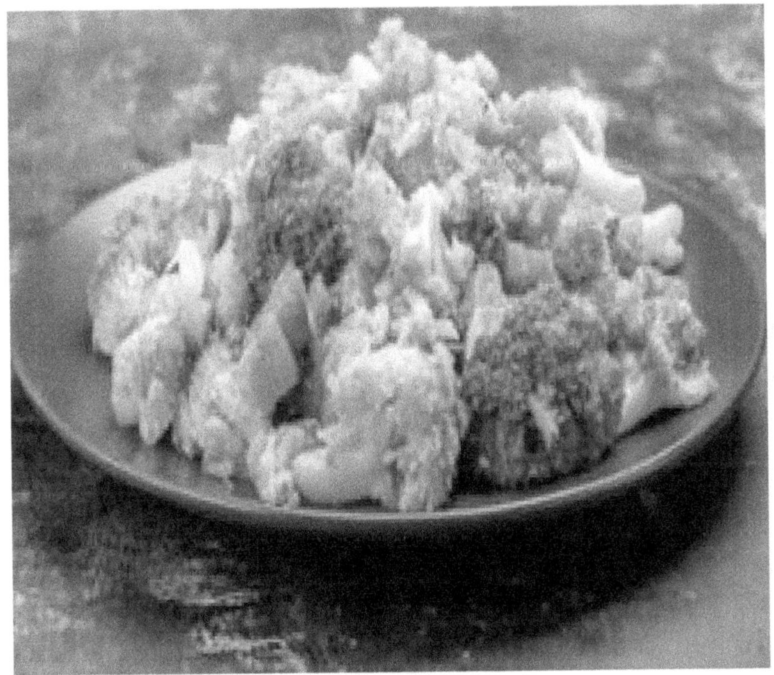

Notes

Your

Observation

CHAPTER 8: DESSERTS DELIGHT

Dark Chocolate Avocado Mousse

Ingredients:

- 2 ripe avocados, peeled and pitted
- 1/2 cup of dark chocolate chips or chopped dark chocolate (70% cocoa or higher)
- 1/4 cup of unsweetened cocoa powder
- 1/4 cup of maple syrup or honey
- 1 teaspoon of vanilla extract
- A pinch of salt
- Fresh berries or mint leaves for garnish (optional)

Preparation:

Melt chocolate:

- Melt the dark chocolate chips or chopped dark chocolate in a heatproof basin. This may be accomplished by putting the bowl over a saucepan of boiling water (double boiler) or by heating in brief bursts in the microwave and stirring in between until smooth. Allow to cool slightly.

Blend avocados:

- In a food processor or blender, mix the peeled and pitted avocados, melted chocolate, unsweetened cocoa powder, maple syrup or honey, vanilla essence, and a pinch of salt.

Blend until smooth:

- Blend the ingredients until smooth and creamy, scraping down the sides of the blender or food processor if necessary. Taste and adjust the sweetness if required.

Chill:

- Transfer the dark chocolate avocado mousse to a dish or serve in individual glasses. Refrigerate for at least 2 hours, or until the mousse is well cold.

Garnish (optional):

- To add a burst of freshness and colour to the Dark Chocolate Avocado Mousse, decorate with fresh berries or mint leaves.

Serve:

- Serve the mousse cooled to enjoy the rich and luscious chocolate flavour.

Enjoy:

- Enjoy this tasty and healthier alternative to typical chocolate mousse, which gets its creamy texture from nutrient-rich avocados.

Nutritional Value (Approximate, per serving):

Calories: 200-250 kcal

Protein: 3g

Fat: 15g (including healthy fats from avocados and dark chocolate)

Carbohydrates: 25g

Dietary Fibre: 7g

Sugar: 15g (from natural sugars in avocados and sweeteners)

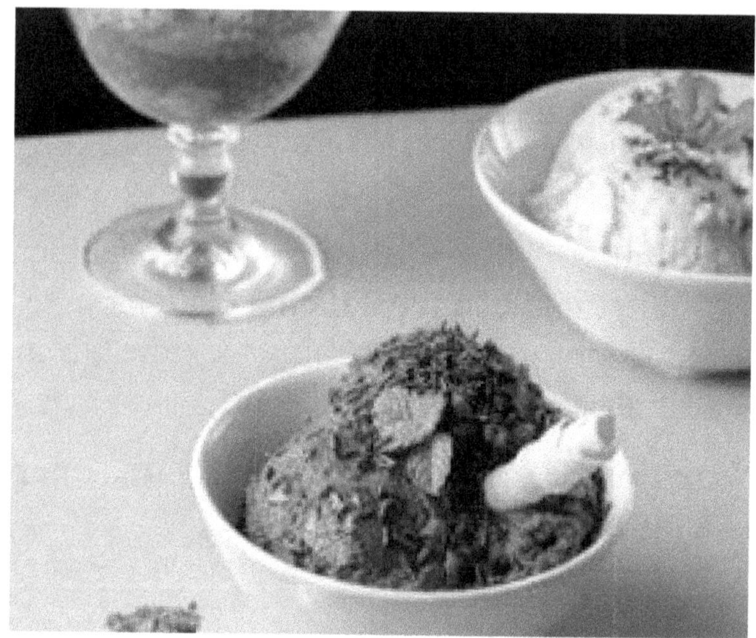

Notes

Your

Observation

Ingredients:

- 1 cup of Greek yogurt (unsweetened)
- 1 cup of mixed berries (strawberries, blueberries, raspberries)
- 1/4 cup of granola (homemade or store-purchased)
- 1 tablespoon honey or maple syrup (optional, for extra sweetness)
- Fresh mint leaves for garnish (optional)

Preparation:

Prepare Greek Yogurt:

- If not previously done, transfer the Greek yoghurt to a bowl. Greek yoghurt provides creaminess and protein to the parfait.

Wash and slice berries:

- Wash the strawberries carefully and slice them if necessary.

Assemble layers:

- In a glass or serving bowl, begin layering the parfait. Start with a teaspoon of Greek yoghurt on the bottom.

Add berries:

- Place a layer of mixed berries on top of the yoghurt. Feel free to mix and match the berries to create different flavours and textures.

Sprinkle granola:

- Sprinkle granola over the fruit. This provides crunch and added nutritional value.

Repeat Layers:

- Repeat the layers until the glass or bowl is full, with a final layer of berries on top.

Drizzle honey (optional):

- If you want to add sweetness, sprinkle honey or maple syrup over the top layer of berries.

Garnish (optional):

- Garnish the Berry and Yoghurt Parfait with fresh mint leaves for a refreshing and visually appealing addition.

Serve immediately:

- Serve the parfait right away to experience the contrasting textures and flavours while the granola is still crispy.

Enjoy:

- This delicious and healthy Berry and Yoghurt Parfait is ideal for a refreshing breakfast, snack, or light dessert.

Nutritional Value (Approximate, per serving):

Calories: 250-300 kcal

Protein: 15g

Fat: 8g (including healthy fats from yogurt and nuts)

Carbohydrates: 35g

Dietary Fiber: 6g

Sugar: 18g (from natural sugars in berries and added sweeteners)

Notes

Your

Observation

Baked Apple Slices with Cinnamon

Ingredients:

- 3-4 average-sized apples, cored and sliced
- 1 tablespoon of melted coconut oil or unsalted butter
- 2 teaspoons of ground cinnamon
- 1 tablespoon of honey or maple syrup (optional, for extra sweetness)
- A pinch of nutmeg (optional)
- Chopped nuts (such as walnuts or pecans) for garnish (optional)
- Greek yogurt or vanilla ice cream for serving (optional)

Preparation:

Preheat the Oven:

- Preheat your oven to 375°F (190°C).

Prepare Apple Slices:

- Core the apples and cut into thin, uniform slices. Leaving the peel on is optional, although it provides more fibre.

Toss with cinnamon:

- In a big mixing bowl, combine the apple slices, melted coconut oil or butter, ground cinnamon, and optional nutmeg until equally covered.

Arrange on a baking sheet:

- Place the cinnamon-coated apple slices in a single layer on a baking sheet lined with parchment paper.

Drizzle with sweetener (optional):

- Drizzle honey or maple syrup over the apple slices to add sweetness. You can adjust the quantity according to your preferences.

Bake in the oven:

- Bake for 20-25 minutes, or until the apples are soft and slightly caramelised, tossing halfway through to ensure equal cooking.

Garnish and serve:

- Once baked, take the apple slices out of the oven. Garnish with chopped nuts if desired.

Serve warm:

- Serve the Baked Apple Slices with Cinnamon warm. They may be eaten on their own or with a dollop of Greek yoghurt or vanilla ice cream.

Enjoy:

- Enjoy easy and delicious treat that accentuates the natural sweetness of apples, complemented by the warmth of cinnamon.

Nutritional Value (Approximate, per serving without toppings):

Calories: 120-150 kcal

Protein: 0.5g

Fat: 3g (including healthy fats from coconut oil or butter)

Carbohydrates: 30g

Dietary Fibre: 5g

Sugar: 20g (from natural sugars in apples and added sweeteners)

Notes

Your

Observation

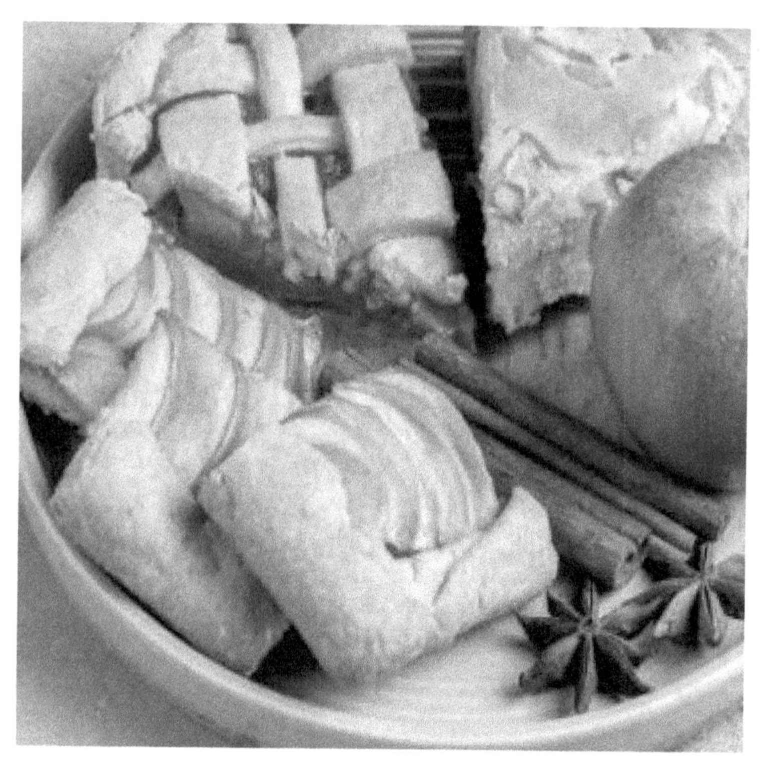

CHAPTER 9: TIPS FOR DINING OUT

Making Heart-Healthy Choices at Restaurants

Choose Grilled or Baked Proteins:

Choose grilled or baked proteins over fried ones. Grilled chicken, fish, and lean meats are healthier alternatives for your heart.

Choose Lean Proteins:

Lean proteins include skinless fowl, fish, beans, lentils, and tofu. These alternatives are low in saturated fat.

Embrace Whole Grains:

Choose entire grains, such as brown rice, quinoa, or whole wheat, as side dishes or meal bases. Whole grains are high in fibre and can improve heart health.

Load Up on Vegetables:

Include a range of colourful vegetables in your meals. Vegetables include vitamins, minerals, and antioxidants that promote heart health.

Mindful Portion Control:

Consider portion amounts. Restaurants frequently provide bigger quantities, which may contribute to overeating. Consider sharing a meal or taking leftovers home.

Reduce Sodium Intake:

To reduce sodium intake, request foods with less added salt and avoid high-sodium products. Ask the chef whether your dish may be prepared with less salt, and use caution with condiments and sauces.

Opt for Healthy Cooking Methods:

Instead of frying, go for healthier cooking methods such as grilling, baking, steaming, or broiling. These methods utilise less oil, lowering the overall fat level of the meal.

Be Cautious of Hidden Fats:

Be wary of hidden fats in dressings, sauces, and toppings. Request sauces on the side, and select vinaigrettes or other heart-healthy dressings.

Choose Heart-Healthy Fats:

Choose heart-healthy fats like olive oil, avocado, and almonds. Consuming these fats in moderation can have a good influence on heart health.

Select Smart Side Dishes:

Instead of fried or creamy sides, go for steamed vegetables, salads with mild dressing, or a side of fruit.

Choose for Water or Unsweetened Beverages:

Instead of sugary beverages, go for water, herbal tea, or other unsweetened options. Limiting additional sugars is helpful to heart health.

Customize Your Order:

Customise your order to meet your specific dietary needs. Many eateries are willing to accept customised orders.

Educate Yourself:

To prepare for a restaurant visit, familiarise yourself with the menu ahead of time. Look for heart-healthy symbols or signs, which some locations offer.

Choose Desserts Wisely:

To control portion sizes, choose fruit-based desserts or share them with others.

By making mindful choices and being aware of the nutritional content of your meal, you can enjoy dining out while prioritizing your heart health.

CHAPTER 10: 10-DAY MEAL PLAN

Breakfast: Greek Yogurt Parfait with Berries and a sprinkle of chia seeds.

Lunch: Quinoa Salad with Grilled Chicken and Mixed Vegetables.

Dinner: Baked Cod with Lemon and Herbs, Steamed Broccoli with Lemon Zest, and Brown Rice.

Breakfast: Energizing Oatmeal with Berries and a handful of almonds.

Lunch: Lentil and Vegetable Soup with a whole-grain roll.

Dinner: Chickpea and Vegetable Stir-Fry with Quinoa.

Breakfast: Almond and Berry Smoothie.

Lunch: Spinach and Salmon Salad with a variety of colorful vegetables.

Dinner: Quinoa and Vegetable Stuffed Peppers, served with a side of mixed greens.

Day 4:

Breakfast: Fresh Fruit Salad with a dollop of Greek yogurt.

Lunch: Sweet Potato and Turkey Chili with a side of whole-grain crackers.

Dinner: Baked Chicken Breast with Roasted Brussels Sprouts and a small serving of sweet potato.

Day 5:

Breakfast: Dark Chocolate Avocado Mousse (small portion).

Lunch: Lentil and Vegetable Wrap with whole-grain tortilla.

Dinner: Grilled Shrimp Skewers with Quinoa and a side of steamed asparagus.

Day 6:

Breakfast: Berry and Yogurt Parfait.

Lunch: Quinoa and Black Bean Salad with a variety of vegetables.

Dinner: Baked Apple Slices with Cinnamon (small portion), Grilled Chicken Breast, and a side of sautéed green beans.

Day 7:

Breakfast: Greek Yogurt with Sliced Banana and a sprinkle of flaxseeds.

Lunch: Chickpea Salad with Cherry Tomatoes, Cucumbers, and Feta cheese.

Dinner: Salmon Fillet with Lemon-Dill Sauce, Quinoa Pilaf, and Roasted Cauliflower.

Day 8:

Breakfast: Almond and Berry Smoothie.

Lunch: Turkey and Avocado Wrap with a whole-grain tortilla.

Dinner: Vegetable and Tofu Stir-Fry with Brown Rice.

Day 9:

Breakfast: Energizing Oatmeal with Sliced Peaches and a sprinkle of walnuts.

Lunch: Quinoa and Vegetable Stuffed Bell Peppers with a side of mixed greens.

Dinner: Baked Cod with Tomato and Olive Relish, Steamed Broccoli, and Quinoa.

Day 10:

Breakfast: Fresh Fruit Salsa with Cinnamon Pita Chips.

Lunch: Lentil and Vegetable Soup with a side of whole-grain bread.

Dinner: Grilled Chicken Breast, Quinoa Salad with Vegetables, and Grilled Zucchini.

CHAPTER 11:
CONCLUSION

Finally, The Complete High Triglyceride Cookbook is an invaluable and powerful resource for anybody who has recently been diagnosed with high triglycerides. As we have studied many dishes and meal plans throughout this cooking guide, it is clear that monitoring and supporting heart health can be a tasty and joyful experience.

The cookbook not only contains a variety of heart-healthy recipes, but it also acts as a resource for making informed dietary decisions. Individuals may proactively manage their triglyceride levels by introducing nutrient-dense foods, lean proteins, and healthy fats into their diet while enjoying enjoyable meals. The emphasis on whole grains, lean meats, and a colourful variety of fruits and vegetables is consistent with a comprehensive approach to cardiovascular health.

Beyond the meals, The Complete High Triglyceride Cookbook promotes a conscious and balanced way of eating. It emphasises portion management, lean cooking techniques, and making informed eating selections. With straightforward directions and easily available supplies, the cookbook appeals to people of all cooking skill levels, instilling confidence and capacity in the kitchen.

Finally, adopting a heart-healthy lifestyle entails more than simply following a series of recipes; it is a commitment to making long-term and good changes. The pathway of controlling triglycerides and boosting heart health is unique to each individual, and The Complete High Triglyceride Cookbook is an invaluable resource.

STAY HEALTHY!

Bonus

MEAL PLANNER
DAILY
DATE
BREAKFAST
NOTES
LUNCH
SNACK
ITEMS LIST
DINNER

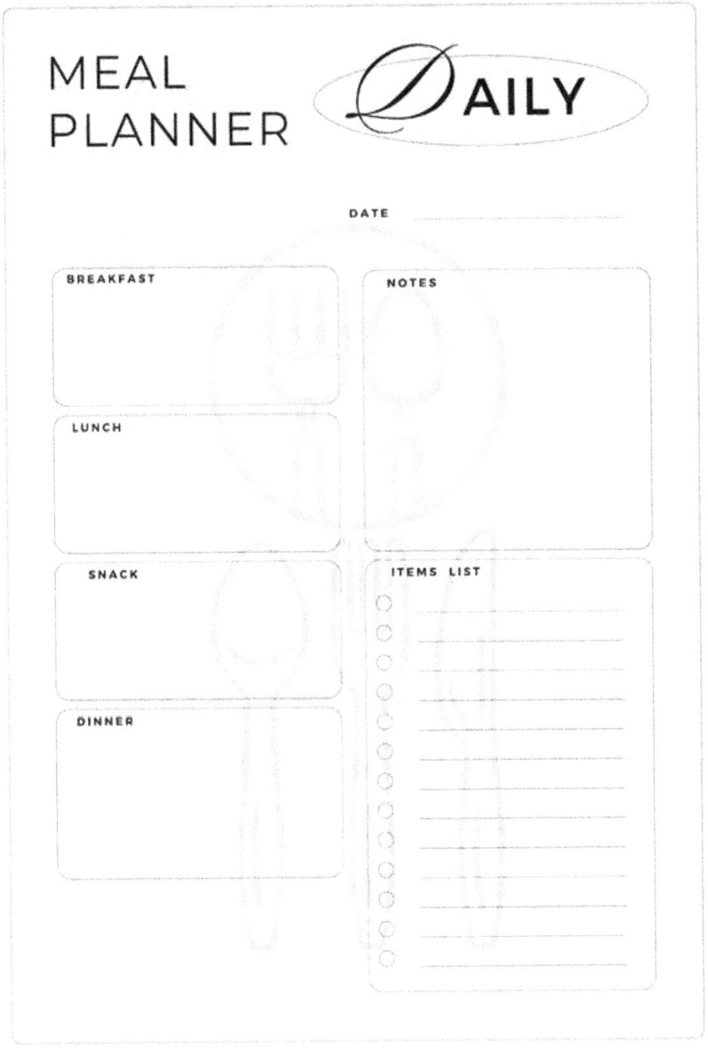

MEAL PLANNER

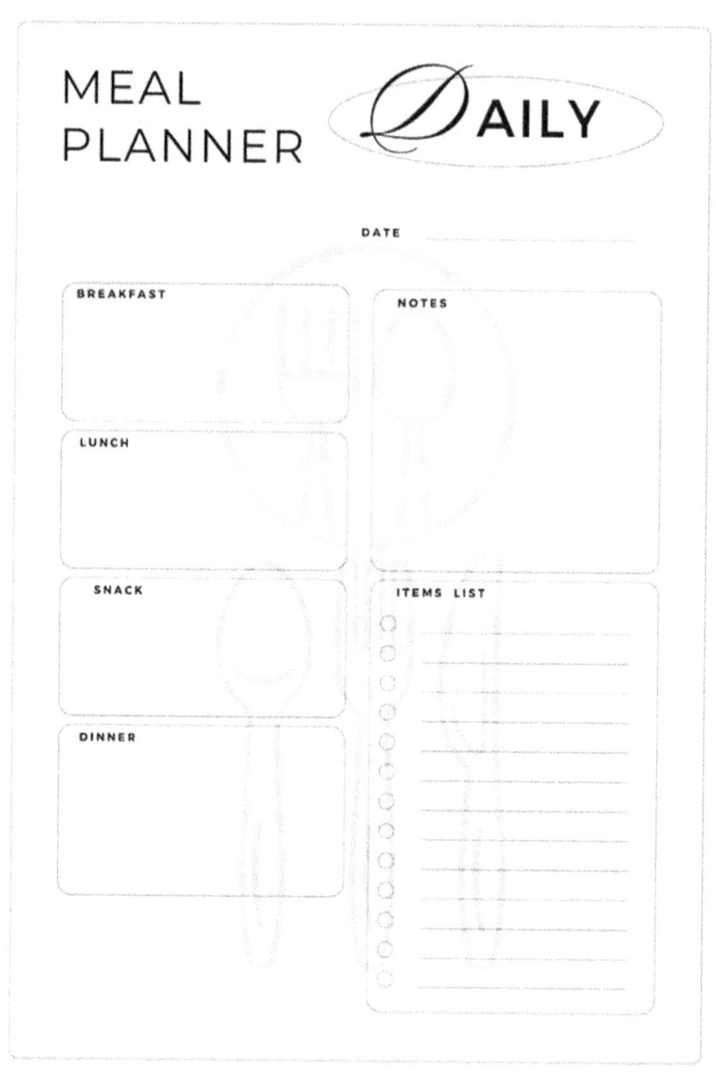

MEAL PLANNER

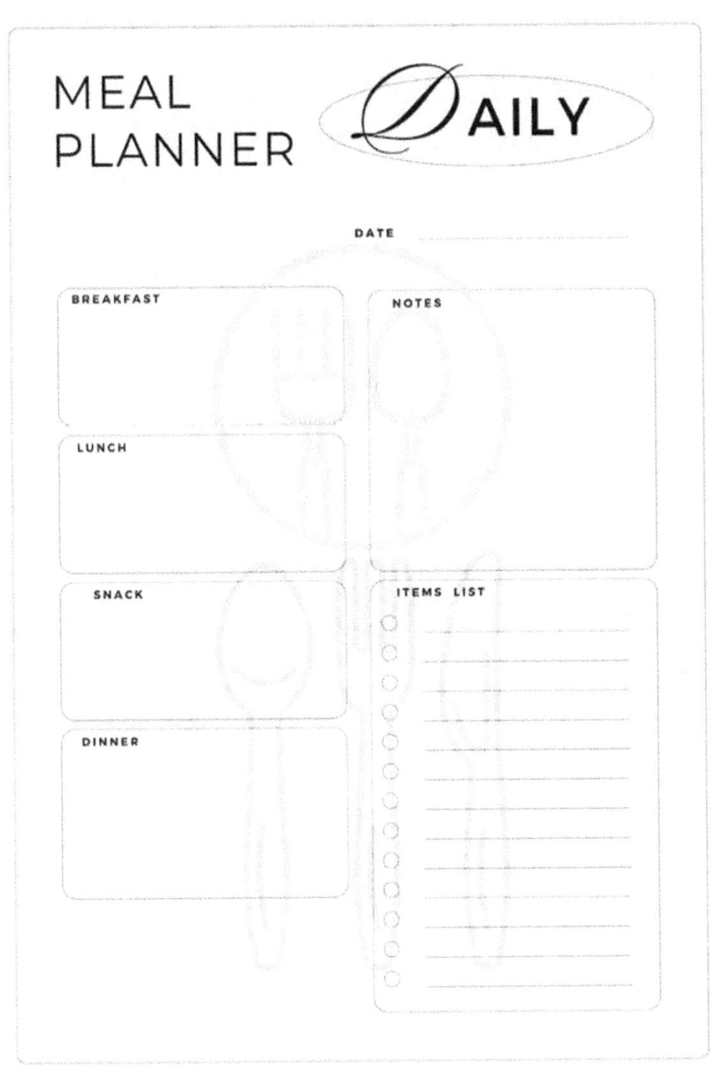

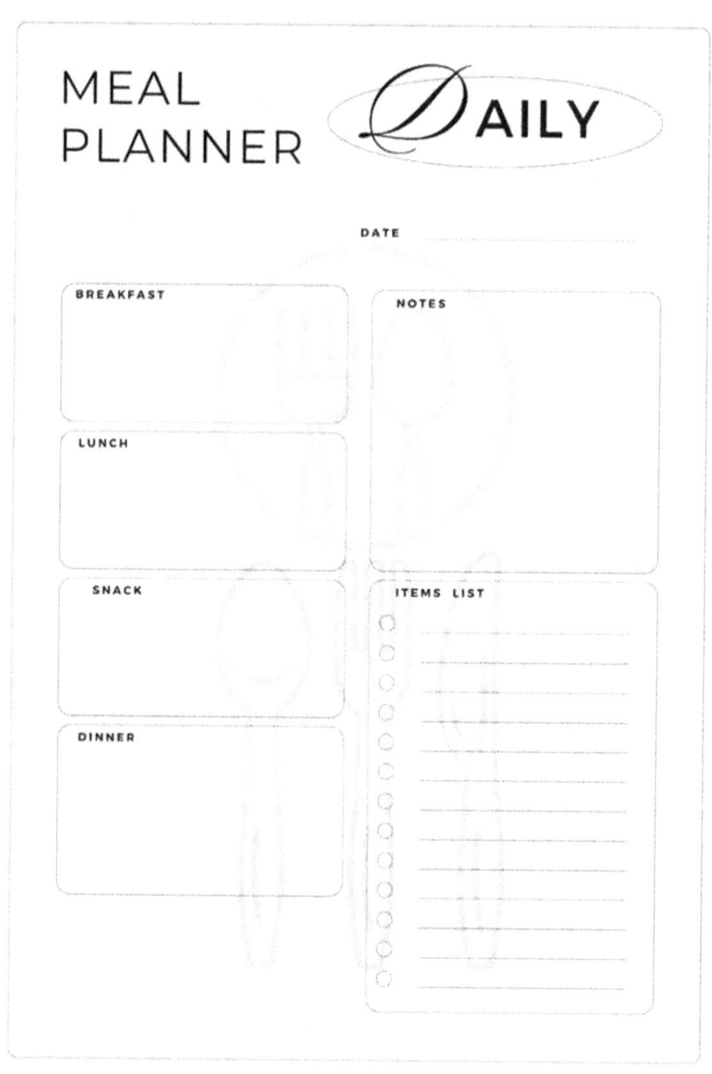

MEAL PLANNER

DAILY

DATE

BREAKFAST

LUNCH

SNACK

DINNER

NOTES

ITEMS LIST

MEAL PLANNER 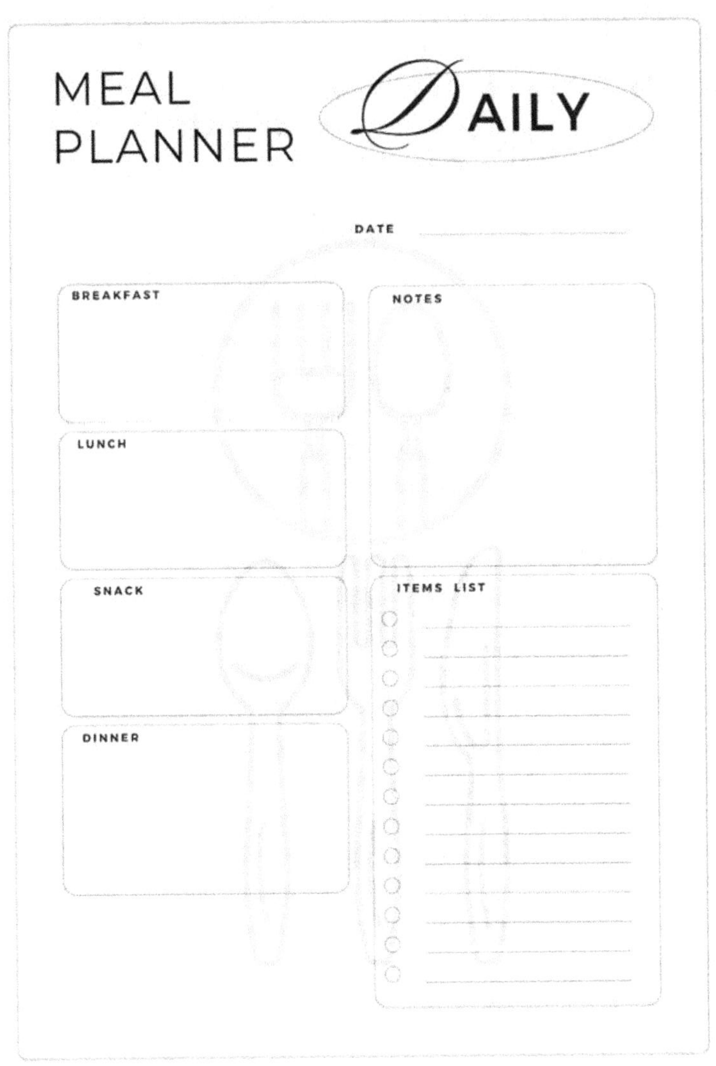

DAILY

DATE

BREAKFAST

LUNCH

SNACK

DINNER

NOTES

ITEMS LIST

MEAL PLANNER

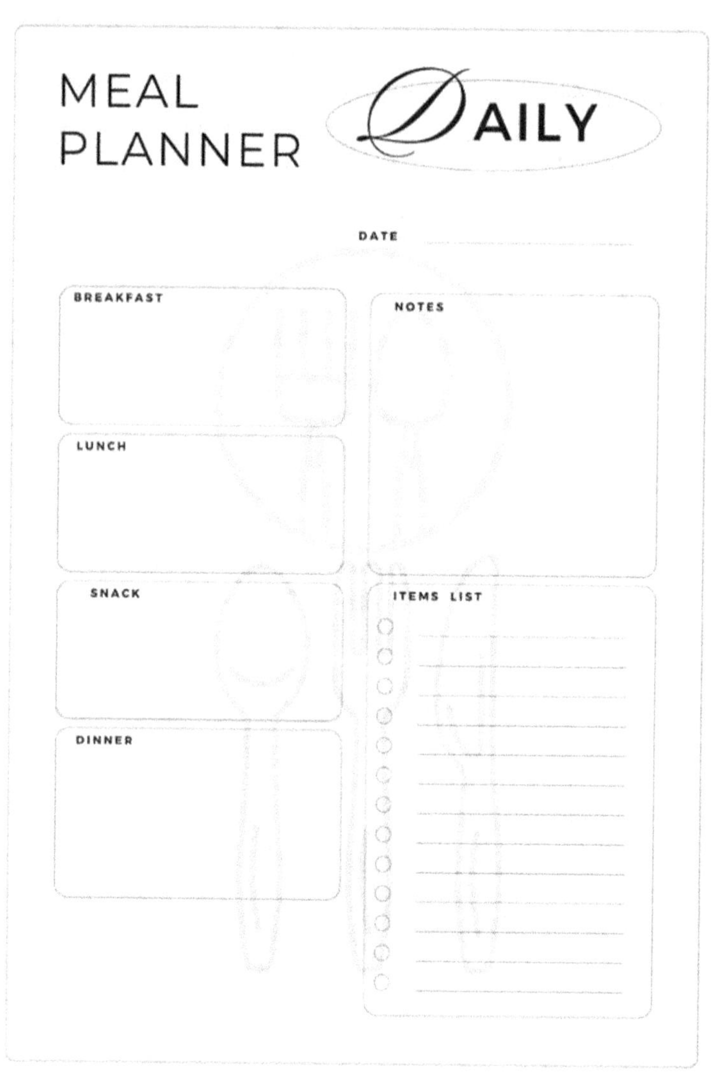

MEAL PLANNER

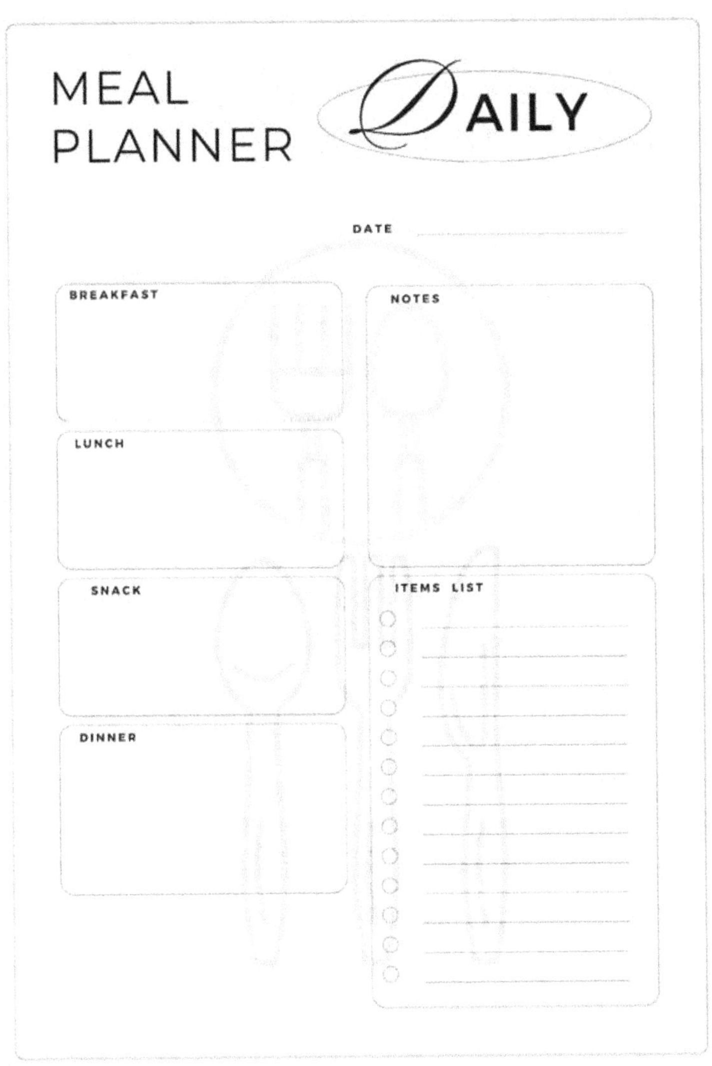

DAILY

DATE

BREAKFAST

LUNCH

SNACK

DINNER

NOTES

ITEMS LIST

MEAL PLANNER

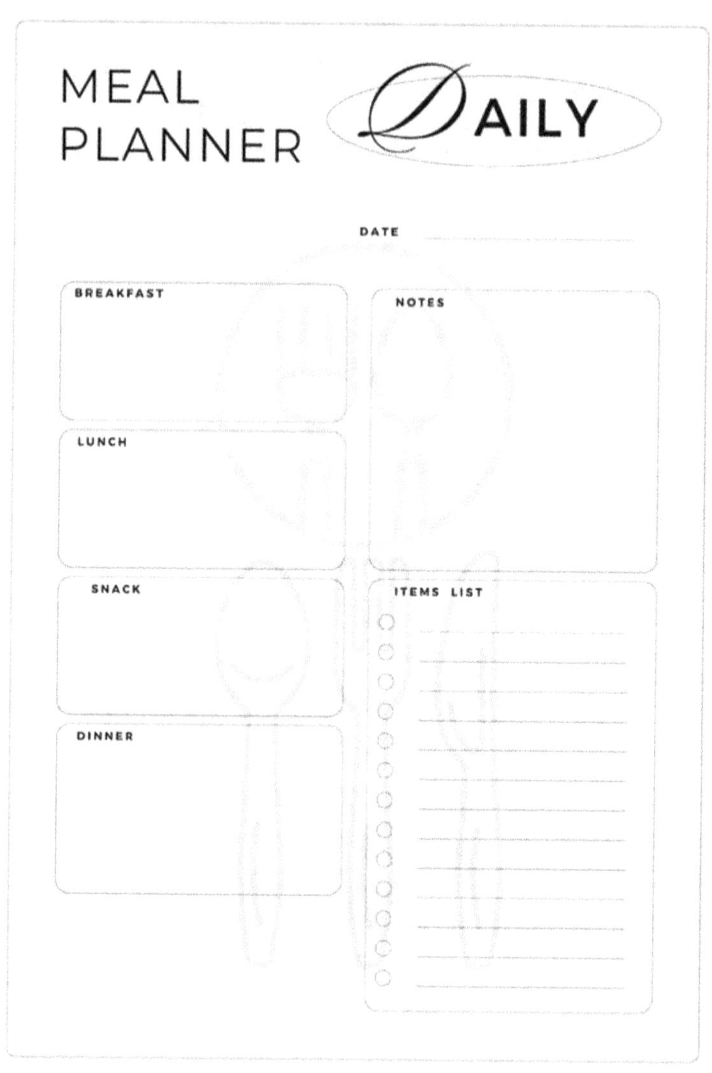

MEAL PLANNER

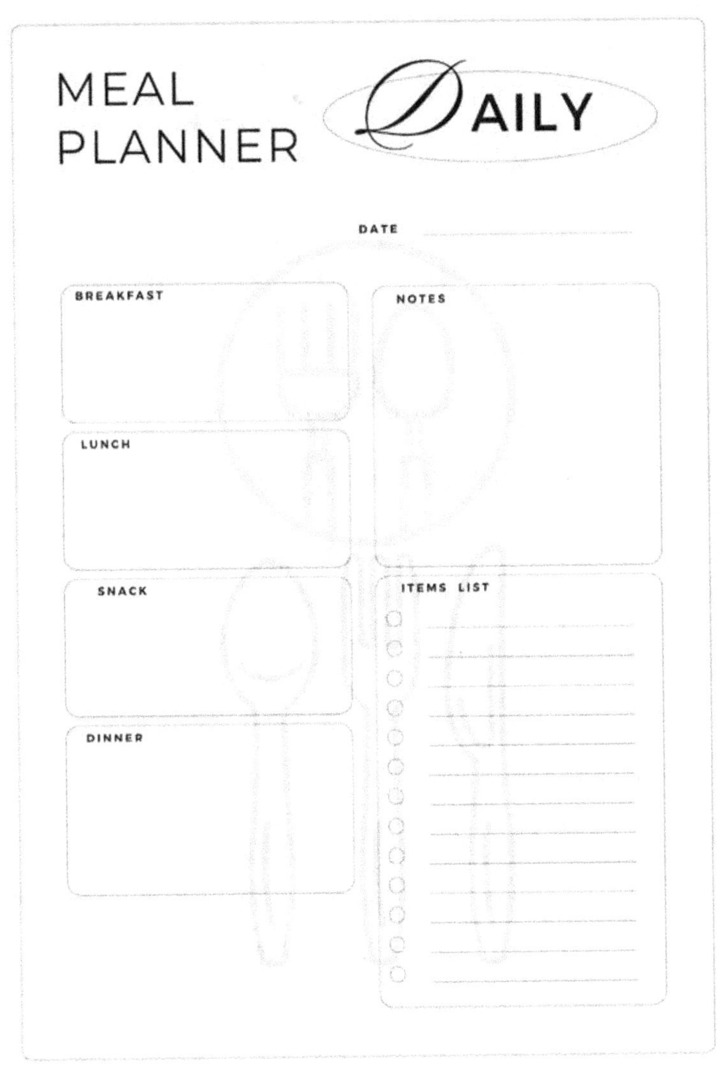

MEAL PLANNER

DAILY

DATE

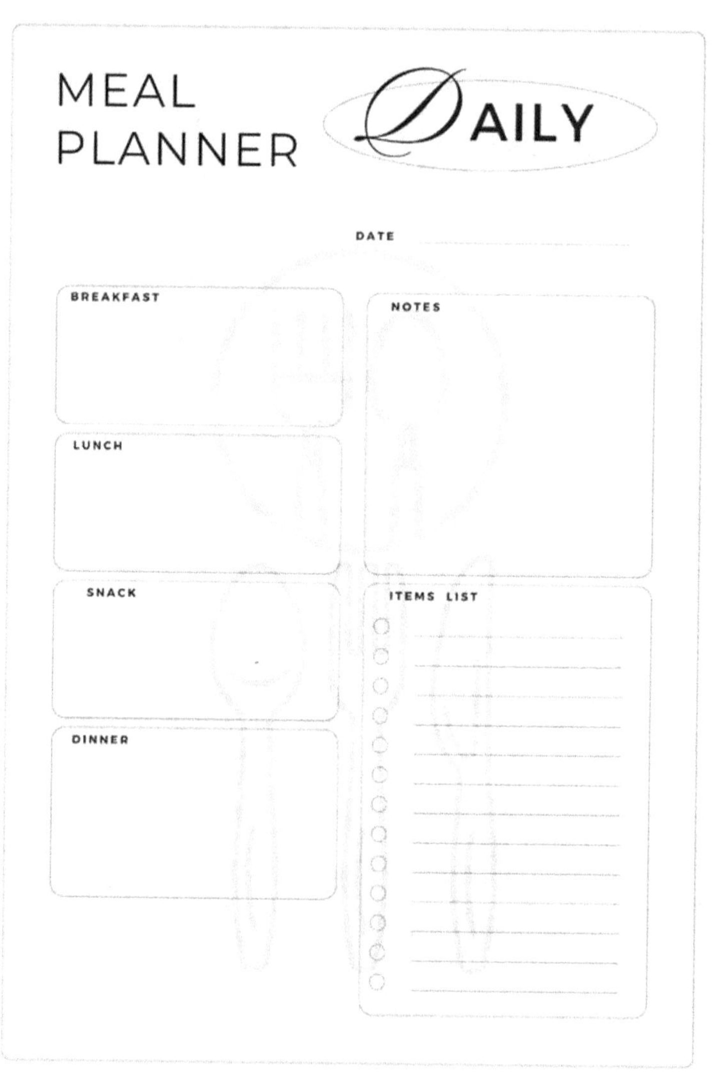

BREAKFAST

LUNCH

SNACK

DINNER

NOTES

ITEMS LIST

9 798880 355037